GoDaWork 4
S.M.A.R.T.I.E.S

Billionaire Veterinarians

Author, Nicshelle Farrow M.A.Ed

Copyright © 2019 Jheryn Renee Smith

All rights reserved.

ISBN:
ISBN-13:

DEDICATION

To every inspired child, student, and parent who wants to have a career in entertainment, dedicate yourself now to learn with the purpose of growing into your career eagerly!

CONTENTS

Acknowledgments   i

1 Veterinarian   Pg #3

2 Veterinarian Work   Pg #7

3 Veterinarian Action   Pg #13

4 Veterinarian Mindset   Pg #20

About the Authors   Pg #34

Author, Nicshelle Farrow

ACKNOWLEDGMENTS

Thank you to all of my family and various supporters that have motivated me and listened to my dreams. In addition, I would like to thank people in advance for providing platforms to motivate other children to become hairstylists and self-published authors.

1 VETERINARIAN

Who wants to be a veterinarian now? I do! I mean business. I've already started doing tasks that a veterinarian does as an adult by washing my dog.

Some people have taken me lightly when I've told them that I'm going to grow up to become a veterinarian. The way I respond to the naysayers is by continuing to visualize myself in my future career as a veterinarian while I play different sports with my family.

Veterinarians are cool. As much as I enjoy helping to take care of my dog with other members of my family, I dream of helping more animals. I've been learning information about snakes, dogs, cats, gerbils, lizards, and horses that are pets. When I become a veterinarian, I plan to help stray animals feel loved too.

Why do you want to become a Veterinarian?

- **Think about the question**
- **Visualize your goal**
- **List details about your response**
- **Share a rationale**
- **Describe your vision**

_____
_____
_____
_____
_____
_____
_____
_____
_____
_____
_____

While you write about your vision, remember to use your experiences to make connections to your new ideas.

_____
_____
_____
_____
_____
_____
_____
_____
_____
_____
_____
_____
_____
_____
_____

2 VETERINARIAN WORK

Based on what I'm learning about business, I plan to not only participate in community projects but spearhead my own projects that support not only pets but other veterinarians.

In the near future, I plan to do more research about the codes and regulations of locations because I plan to own a veterinarian business. It will not only support my position as a community liaison and be able to provide employment. It will be an astronomical opportunity for me to be able to learn more about being a veterinarian from doing an internship before I'm able to go to college.

Yes, I'm working on positioning myself already toward making more money than someone that doesn't have a college education as I grow and develop into a billionaire.

How do you plan to learn more about the business of being a Veterinarian?

- **Think about the question**
- **Visualize your goal**
- **List details about your response**
- **Share a rationale**
- **Describe your vision**

_____
_____
_____
_____
_____
_____
_____
_____
_____
_____

While you write about your vision, remember to use your experiences to make connections to your new ideas.

_____
_____
_____
_____
_____
_____
_____
_____
_____
_____
_____
_____
_____
_____

Author, Nicshelle Farrow

3 VETERINARIAN ACTION

Drama is what I've been watching in various places. Pets and stray animals help people to combat stress that surrounds them. Imagine the following excerpt from a movie:

Co-Worker: Did you see that dog running?
Community Representative: Please don't call the dog pound, call the Veterinarian!
Pet: Who is Veterinarian and where is Veterinarian?
Surveillance Monitor: Let me call, Veterinarian.

Co-Worker: Why is Veterinarian walking that dog?
Community Representative: Goodness!
Pet: Help me Veterinarian! I'm on a food mission.
Surveillance Monitor: That dog is hungry.

Co-Worker: Hello, Veterinarian you're off work.
The Veterinarian: Now, I'm not.

Pet: Veterinarian must be awesome!
Surveillance Monitor: Where is she going to find a home for this dog? Her community must have 100's of loving homes awaiting a dog under Veterinarian the Veterinarian's care.

What will your lifestyle be like as a Veterinarian?

- Think about the question
- Visualize your goal
- List details about your response
- Share a rationale
- Describe your vision

_____

_____

_____

_____
_____
_____
_____
_____

While you write about your vision, remember to use your experiences to make connections to your new ideas.

_____
_____
_____
_____
_____

4 VETERINARIAN MINDSET

There is a plethora of information in the in the world about veterinarians, pets, stray animals, and their habitats. My focus is to help provide as many locations of 24 hour animal daycares so that even non-profit organizations can contribute money to prevent lack of care for animals.

This year, it's really interesting that I want to become a veterinarian when I state my career goal. My mind is made up. I've been wearing clothes that appeal to the eye that I may already be a veterinarian. My focus on drama is intrigued by the other medical shows that I watch.

From what I've been experiencing as a student, I believe I'm equipped and more than prepared to become a phenomenal veterinarian as soon as possible.

What will motivate you when you encounter challenges as a Veterinarian?

- **Think about the question**
- **Visualize your goal**
- **List details about your response**
- **Share a rationale**
- **Describe your vision**

_____
_____
_____
_____
_____
_____
_____
_____
_____

ABOUT THE AUTHORS

Nicshelle is a networking machine. She networks under many hats that she wears as a filmmaker, photographer, actress, comedian, radio and red carpet events' host, motivational speaker, author, scriptwriter, advertisement consultant, film, and literary editor.

EDUCATION & CREDENTIALS

M.A.Ed University of Phoenix, Henderson, Nevada 2008

B.A. University of Dominguez Hills, Carson, California 2001

A.A. Community College of Southern Nevada, Las Vegas, Nevada 1992

Pi Lambda Theta, National Education Society

www.ingramcontent.com/pod-product-compliance
Lightning Source LLC
Chambersburg PA
CBHW030551220526

45463CB00007B/3062